CHART TO SAVE YOUR RN LICENSE

The Nurse's Blueprint for Safe, Clear, and Accurate Documentation

FLORENCE CLARA

© 2024 by FLORENCE CLARA. All rights reserved.

No part of this book may be reproduced or utilized in any form or by any means, electronic or mechanical, including photocopying, recording, or by any information storage and retrieval system, without permission in writing from the publisher.

First Edition 2024

Published by FLORENCE CLARA

DISCLAIMER

This book is intended as an informational guide written by a nurse, for nurses, to enhance understanding and encourage compliance with nursing protocols. It is not a substitute for official nursing laws or facility guidelines. Always follow the specific legal requirements and standards of your state and workplace.

Table Of Content

INTRODUCTION 5

CHAPTER 1 7

Introduction to the Importance of Proper Charting 7

CHAPTER 2 11

Legal and Ethical Standards in Nursing Documentation 11

CHAPTER 3 16

Fundamentals of Clear and Concise Charting 16

CHAPTER 4 21

Documenting Patient Care: What to Include and What to Avoid 21

CHAPTER 5 27

Charting in High-Stress Situations: Emergencies and Critical Care . 27

CHAPTER 6 34

Electronic Health Records (EHR): Navigating Modern Charting Tools 34

Chapter 7 40

Protecting Your License: Documenting Incidents, Errors, and Near Misses 41

Chapter 8 48

Audit-Proofing Your Documentation: Preparing for Investigations . 48

Chapter 9 55

Defensive Documentation: Protecting Yourself in Litigation 55

Chapter 10 61

Continuous Improvement: Ongoing Education and Best Practices in Documentation 61

CONCLUSION 68

Bonus Tips for Charting on a Typical Shift 68

INTRODUCTION

Let me take you back to a moment in my career that changed everything. I had been a registered nurse for nearly 15 years, confident in my abilities and committed to patient care. But one afternoon, I found myself sitting in a meeting room, palms sweating, facing an unexpected audit of my patient records. A routine chart entry I had completed in a rush during a particularly chaotic shift was being scrutinized for its accuracy. My heart sank. That one moment of oversight, a rushed charting mistake, now had the potential to jeopardize my entire career—my RN license.

Like many nurses, I took pride in my work, but I hadn't fully appreciated the true value of my RN license until it was on the line. This credential isn't just a formality; it's the foundation of our profession. It allows us to legally practice, to care for others, and to serve our communities. Without it, years of education, training, and experience become irrelevant, and the career we've worked so hard to build can vanish in an instant.

An RN license symbolizes more than just a qualification—it embodies trust. Patients trust that when they're in our care, they're being looked after by professionals who are skilled, ethical, and regulated. Hospitals and healthcare organizations depend on licensed nurses to uphold the highest standards of care. The license ensures that we're held accountable to both our patients and the profession itself. It's the key to our career, and without it, we can't do what we're trained to do: provide compassionate and effective care.

But as I learned that day, protecting your license is about more than just clinical competency—it's about how you document every aspect of your work. Charting, often viewed as a tedious task, is actually one of the most critical components of nursing. Those entries, time-stamped and archived, serve as legal records that may be called upon in audits, investigations, or even court cases. A simple mistake, an omission, or an unclear note can place your entire career in jeopardy.

In my case, that experience was a wake-up call. I realized that no matter how skilled we are as nurses, our license is only as safe as our documentation. It was this lesson that inspired me to write this book—because I don't want any other nurse to face the stress, fear, or uncertainty that I did. I want you to have the tools to not only care for your patients but to protect your license every step of the way.

Throughout this book, I will share insights, strategies, and best practices for mastering the art of documentation. You'll learn how to chart efficiently and accurately, how to avoid common mistakes, and how to safeguard your professional future. Whether you're a new nurse just starting your career or a seasoned professional, the lessons here are critical to keeping your license—and your career—secure.

Your RN license is your most valuable asset. Without it, the career you've worked so hard for could be at risk. Let's make sure that never happens. Join me as we explore the essential steps to charting that will protect both your patients and your professional future.

CHAPTER 1

Introduction to the Importance of Proper Charting

As nurses, we are entrusted with the care and well-being of our patients. Our responsibilities go far beyond the bedside, as the care we provide must be captured accurately and thoroughly in our documentation—commonly referred to as "charting." While charting can sometimes feel like a routine part of the job, it is actually one of the most critical aspects of nursing practice. Proper charting is not just a matter of professional diligence, but also a safeguard for both patients and nurses. It serves as an essential legal document and professional record that can be the determining factor in many legal and clinical situations.

Charting: More Than Just Paperwork

To the untrained eye, charting might appear to be a mundane part of nursing—a necessary evil in a fast-paced healthcare environment. However, the reality is that charting is much more than mere paperwork. It is the structured documentation of the care you provide, a detailed log that communicates vital patient information across healthcare teams and serves as the foundation of future patient care decisions.

Every entry you make in a patient's record not only reflects the nursing care provided but also offers legal proof of the actions taken and the clinical judgments made. This is particularly important in cases where outcomes are less than ideal or when questions arise about the care provided. In such cases, the medical record is often the only solid evidence available, and the quality of the documentation can determine whether or not the nurse's actions were appropriate and legally defensible.

Why Proper Charting is Vital to Patient Care

Accurate charting directly impacts the quality of patient care. Healthcare is a team effort, and nurses often hand off patients to other professionals. If your charting is unclear, incomplete, or inaccurate, you run the risk of compromising patient safety. Proper documentation ensures continuity of care, allowing other healthcare professionals to understand exactly what has been done, what is planned, and what the patient's current condition is.

Take, for example, a nurse who neglects to document that a patient received a medication. The next nurse, not seeing the documentation, might administer the same medication again, potentially leading to a dangerous overdose. Alternatively, failure to record a patient's allergic reaction could result in the patient being exposed to the same allergen again, with potentially fatal consequences. Proper documentation prevents these kinds of mistakes and ensures that patient care is safe, consistent, and informed.

The Consequences of Poor Documentation

Inaccurate or incomplete charting can lead to a range of negative consequences, both for the patient and the nurse. For the patient, poor documentation can result in incorrect treatments, delayed care, or even harmful medical errors. For the nurse, the repercussions can be even more severe. Nursing boards and courts routinely rely on documentation when evaluating claims of negligence or malpractice. A chart that is incomplete or vague can easily be interpreted as a failure to provide adequate care, even if the nurse did everything correctly. The chart is the nurse's primary defense in such cases, and poor documentation leaves a nurse vulnerable to legal and professional consequences.

Consider a scenario where a patient files a complaint against a nurse for negligence, and the nurse's charting lacks essential details about the care provided. In the absence of clear documentation, it becomes difficult to prove that the nurse acted in accordance with the standard of care. In these situations, even if the nurse provided excellent care, the lack of proper documentation could lead to disciplinary action, including suspension or revocation of the nurse's license. In some cases, poor charting can even lead to lawsuits and costly legal battles, potentially tarnishing the nurse's professional reputation.

Charting as a Legal and Professional Safeguard

Beyond being a clinical tool, charting is a critical legal safeguard for nurses. In a profession where the stakes are high and errors can lead to severe consequences, documentation serves as both a record of care and a legal document. In many malpractice cases, the medical record is the primary piece of evidence. Clear, comprehensive documentation can exonerate a nurse by showing that appropriate care was provided, while poor or incomplete documentation can leave a nurse vulnerable to accusations of neglect or misconduct.

For instance, when an adverse event occurs, the first thing an investigating board or legal team will examine is the patient's medical record. They will look for specific details about what actions were taken, what assessments were made, and what the nurse's rationale was for those decisions. A well-documented chart will clearly demonstrate the nurse's clinical judgment and decision-making process, providing a defense against claims of negligence. On the other hand, missing or vague information in the record can lead to the assumption that important aspects of care were overlooked, even if that was not the case.

Real-Life Consequences: A Lesson from Experience

I once witnessed a colleague, an experienced nurse, face a situation where poor charting nearly cost her career. After a hectic shift in a critical care unit, she inadvertently failed to document a vital reassessment of a patient who had received medication for a serious cardiac condition. The patient later experienced complications, and during an audit, her incomplete charting became a focal point of concern. Although she had provided the necessary care, the missing documentation led to an investigation by the nursing board. It was a wake-up call for all of us—documentation is not just a task to be completed, it's our primary defense in safeguarding our license and career.

Setting the Stage for the Rest of the Book

This book will guide you through the intricacies of charting, showing you how to document in a way that protects not only your patients but also your career. In the following chapters, you will learn how to master clear, concise, and legally sound documentation, how to navigate complex situations like incidents or emergencies, and how to safeguard your RN license through best practices in charting. As you proceed, you will understand that while charting may sometimes feel like a chore, it is your greatest ally in delivering excellent patient care and protecting the license you've worked so hard to obtain.

Proper documentation is the foundation of nursing practice, patient safety, and legal protection. By mastering this skill, you not only ensure that your patients receive the highest quality of care but also secure your own professional future.

CHAPTER 2

Legal and Ethical Standards in Nursing Documentation

As a nurse, you are held to the highest legal and ethical standards when it comes to documenting patient care. Documentation is not just a professional requirement but also a legal obligation that ensures patient safety and protects both nurses and healthcare organizations from legal liabilities. Understanding the legal frameworks and ethical principles that guide nursing documentation is critical for maintaining the integrity of your practice and protecting your RN license.

Legal Standards Governing Nursing Documentation

Health Insurance Portability and Accountability Act (HIPAA)

One of the most important regulations governing nursing documentation is the Health Insurance Portability and Accountability Act (HIPAA). HIPAA was enacted in 1996 to protect patient privacy and secure sensitive health information. Nurses are required by law to ensure that patient records are kept confidential and are only shared with individuals who are authorized to access that information, such as other healthcare providers directly involved in the patient's care.

HIPAA violations can result in severe penalties, including fines and disciplinary actions, even if the breach was unintentional. For example, if a nurse leaves a chart open on a computer screen where unauthorized individuals can view it, this could be considered a violation of patient privacy. Failing to safeguard patient information in documentation can not only harm patients but also lead to legal consequences for the nurse, such as termination, loss of licensure, or lawsuits.

State Nursing Practice Acts

Each state has its own Nursing Practice Act, which outlines the legal scope of practice for nurses, including documentation requirements. These laws specify what must be included in nursing records and mandate that documentation be timely, accurate, and complete. Failing to follow these guidelines can result in charges of professional misconduct and, in severe cases, can lead to the suspension or revocation of your nursing license.

For example, a nurse who neglects to chart critical information, such as a patient's adverse reaction to medication, may be found in violation of their state's Nursing Practice Act. This can result in legal consequences and may jeopardize the nurse's ability to practice.

The Joint Commission

The Joint Commission, an independent, non-profit organization that accredits healthcare organizations in the United States, sets standards for patient care, including documentation practices. Nurses working in accredited institutions must follow the Joint Commission's guidelines, which emphasize the importance of accurate, complete, and legible documentation. Failing to meet these standards can lead to citations against the healthcare facility, which may result in financial penalties or loss of accreditation.

Ethical Principles in Nursing Documentation

In addition to legal obligations, nurses must follow a strict code of ethics when documenting patient care. These ethical principles serve as the foundation for maintaining professionalism, integrity, and trust in healthcare.

Honesty and Integrity

Honesty is one of the core ethical principles in nursing documentation. When charting, nurses must ensure that every entry is a truthful and accurate reflection of the care provided. This means recording exactly what was done, when it was done, and why it was done. Any attempt to alter or falsify documentation—whether to cover a mistake or to give the impression that care was provided when it wasn't—is a serious ethical breach.

For example, a nurse who accidentally administers the wrong medication but fails to document the error in an attempt to avoid reprimand is not only violating ethical standards but is also putting their license at risk. In the event of an investigation, altered or missing documentation is often seen as an admission of wrongdoing, which can lead to disciplinary action, termination, or legal proceedings.

Accountability

Nurses are accountable for the care they provide, and this accountability extends to the documentation of that care. Every entry a nurse makes in a patient's record should reflect their professional judgment and adherence to standards of care. If something goes wrong, the chart will serve as evidence of the nurse's actions—or inactions—and will be used to determine whether the nurse met the expected standard of care.

Consider a scenario in which a nurse fails to document a critical change in a patient's condition, such as a sudden drop in blood pressure. If the patient later deteriorates and the documentation does not reflect timely interventions, the nurse could be held accountable for failing to recognize and act on the change in condition. This lack of accountability in documentation could result in legal repercussions, professional discipline, or loss of licensure.

Objectivity and Non-bias

Nursing documentation must always be objective and free of personal bias or subjective opinions. The role of a nurse is to provide factual, evidence-based care, and this should be reflected in the chart. Subjective comments, assumptions, or derogatory remarks have no place in nursing documentation and can undermine the nurse's professionalism.

For instance, writing "The patient was rude and non-cooperative" is subjective and unprofessional. A more appropriate and objective entry would be "The patient declined medication at 9:00 AM and stated they were feeling better." This type of entry provides factual information without making assumptions about the patient's behavior or intent.

Real-Life Consequences of Documentation Errors

The legal and ethical principles of documentation are not just theoretical—they have real-world implications. Documentation errors can lead to serious legal disputes and disciplinary actions that can jeopardize a nurse's license and career.

Legal Disputes

Documentation errors are one of the leading causes of malpractice claims. When a lawsuit is filed, the medical record is often the primary piece of evidence used to determine whether the nurse met the standard of care. Inconsistent, incomplete, or incorrect documentation can give the appearance that care was substandard, even if the nurse's actions were appropriate.

For example, in a legal case where a nurse failed to document a patient's deteriorating condition in a timely manner, the court ruled that the nurse was negligent, even though she had been providing care. The absence of proper documentation made it impossible for the nurse to prove that she had recognized and responded to the patient's needs.

Disciplinary Actions

Beyond lawsuits, documentation errors can result in disciplinary actions from licensing boards. A nurse who consistently fails to document patient care accurately may be subject to investigation by their state's board of nursing. Depending on the severity of the documentation errors, the board may impose sanctions, such as fines, mandatory retraining, or in severe cases, license suspension or revocation.

For instance, a nurse who fails to document an incident where a patient fell may face disciplinary action if the fall later leads to a serious injury. The absence of documentation makes it difficult to determine what care was provided after the fall and whether the nurse acted appropriately

How Legal and Ethical Standards Protect Nurses and Patients

Legal regulations like HIPAA and state Nursing Practice Acts, along with ethical principles of honesty, integrity, and accountability, are in place to protect both nurses and patients. Following these standards in your documentation helps ensure patient safety, fosters trust in the healthcare system, and protects your RN license from legal and professional risks.

As you proceed through this book, remember that every chart entry is not just a reflection of your patient care—it's a reflection of your professional integrity. Proper documentation is your best defense against legal disputes and the key to safeguarding your nursing license.

CHAPTER 3

Fundamentals of Clear and Concise Charting

Writing nursing notes may feel routine, but it is one of the most critical aspects of your role as a nurse. Accurate documentation not only ensures continuity of care for patients, but it also serves as your professional defense should your actions ever be questioned. Clear, concise, and effective nursing notes help avoid misunderstandings, protect you from legal consequences, and improve overall communication within the healthcare team.

In this chapter, we'll focus on practical strategies you can use to document efficiently while adhering to legal and ethical standards.

The Importance of Clarity in Documentation

Clear communication is the foundation of good nursing documentation. Nursing notes should provide enough detail to paint a complete picture of the patient's condition, the care provided, and the outcomes of interventions. Clarity ensures that anyone who reads the notes—whether it's another nurse, a physician, or a legal team—can understand exactly what happened and why.

Here's a real-world example of poor documentation:

Poor Documentation Example:

"Patient seems better today. No complaints."

This entry is vague and lacks detail. What does "better" mean? Were vital signs taken? Was the patient assessed for pain? This entry provides little useful information to guide future care or defend the nurse's actions in the event of a dispute.

Now, let's compare it to a clearer version:

Better Documentation Example:

"Patient reports no pain at 9:00 AM. Vital signs stable: BP 120/80, HR 72, SpO2 98% on room air. Ambulated with assistance for 15 minutes without shortness of breath or fatigue."

This entry provides concrete data, including the patient's report, objective measurements (vital signs), and a description of the intervention (ambulation) and its outcome. It's clear, concise, and paints a complete picture of the patient's condition

Avoiding Vague Language

One of the most common pitfalls in nursing documentation is the use of vague language. Words like "appears," "seems," or "looks" should be avoided because they are subjective and open to interpretation. Instead, focus on objective observations that can be backed up with measurable data.

Vague:

"Patient seems uncomfortable."

Better:

"Patient grimacing, clutching abdomen. Reports pain as 8/10 at 10:00 AM. Administered 5 mg morphine IV as ordered."

The second entry is specific, factual, and detailed. It describes the patient's behavior (grimacing, clutching abdomen), the subjective report (8/10 pain), and the nurse's intervention (morphine administration). This level of detail ensures that the note is clear and defensible.

Limiting Medical Jargon

While it's easy to fall into the habit of using medical jargon, especially in fast-paced settings, it's important to remember that not everyone who reads your documentation may be familiar with specialized terms. Other healthcare professionals, legal personnel, or even patients themselves may review the chart at some point. Using clear, everyday language helps ensure that your notes can be understood by all parties involved.

For example:

Too much jargon:

"Pt desatted post-extubation, requiring reintubation at 20:00."

Better:

"Patient's oxygen saturation dropped to 85% after extubation at 19:50. Reintubated at 20:00 to maintain the airway and increase oxygenation."

The second entry avoids unnecessary jargon, providing a clear explanation of what happened in a way that is understandable to all readers.

Objectivity: Keeping Personal Opinions Out

Nursing documentation must always be objective, focusing on observable facts rather than personal opinions or emotions. Your role as a nurse is to provide professional, unbiased care, and this should be reflected in your notes.

Inappropriate Opinion:

"Patient is being difficult and refuses to cooperate with care."

Better:

"Patient refused to take prescribed medication at 9:30 AM, stating they felt nauseated."

The second entry removes any bias and simply states the facts: the patient refused medication and gave a reason. It leaves out the nurse's subjective interpretation, which could be seen as unprofessional or even inflammatory.

Techniques for Concise Charting

While it's important to be thorough, there's no need to write a novel in each entry. The key is to document the essential facts without unnecessary details. Being concise means including relevant information that communicates the patient's condition and your actions clearly.

Follow these guidelines to write concise, yet effective notes:

Stick to the facts: Describe what you observed, what the patient reported, and what interventions were performed.

Use abbreviations sparingly: Only use approved medical abbreviations, and avoid using too many in one note to prevent confusion.

Follow the SOAP or DAR format: Structured formats like SOAP (Subjective, Objective, Assessment, Plan) or DAR (Data, Action, Response) can help keep your notes organized and concise without leaving out important details.

Example using **SOAP** format:

S: Patient reports chest pain at 2:00 PM, describes it as "sharp" and "stabbing," rates pain 7/10.

O: BP 150/90, HR 110, RR 22, SpO2 96%. Skin pale and diaphoretic.

A: Acute chest pain, possible cardiac event.

P: Notified MD, administered nitroglycerin 0.4 mg SL per order. Patient to remain on bed rest until reassessed.

Using a structured format like this ensures that your documentation is complete, organized, and easy to read.

How Clear Documentation Protects Your License

Clear, concise, and factual documentation serves as a legal record of the care you provided. In any situation where your actions are questioned—whether by a supervisor, a court, or a licensing board—your notes will be used as evidence of what you did (or didn't) do. Vague, incomplete, or inaccurate documentation can lead to misunderstandings, miscommunication among healthcare providers, and in the worst cases, legal action against you.

For instance, consider a situation where a patient's condition deteriorates overnight, and the nursing notes are incomplete. If the next shift's nurse has no clear understanding of the patient's baseline condition or previous care, critical information could be missed, leading to delays in treatment. Worse, if the case goes to court, the lack of documentation could imply negligence, even if you provided appropriate care.

Good documentation protects not only the patient's well-being but also your professional integrity. By providing clear, objective, and concise notes, you ensure that your work is transparent and defensible, safeguarding both your practice and your RN license.

Writing effective nursing notes is a skill that takes practice, but it's one of the most important aspects of protecting both your patients and your career. Clear, concise, and objective documentation ensures that your actions are understood, your patients receive the best possible care, and your professional record is safeguarded. By avoiding vague language, medical jargon, and personal opinions, and by focusing on the facts, you can write notes that stand up to any level of scrutiny, whether by your colleagues or by legal professionals.

In the next chapter, we'll delve into the specifics of documenting patient care, including what to include and what to avoid to ensure your notes are comprehensive and accurate.

CHAPTER 4

Documenting Patient Care: What to Include and What to Avoid

As nurses, we know that documentation is a core responsibility of our daily practice. It forms the foundation of patient care, creates a vital communication link between members of the healthcare team, and serves as a legal record of everything we do. But knowing what to include, what to avoid, and how to balance thoroughness without overwhelming details can be challenging. In this chapter, we'll dive into the essential components that should always be included in nursing documentation, and explore the potential pitfalls of over-documentation and under-documentation.

Essential Components of Daily Nursing Records

Effective documentation is about striking a balance between providing sufficient detail and ensuring clarity. The following are the key components that must be documented daily to ensure that the patient's care is clearly communicated to other healthcare providers and to protect yourself from legal consequences.

1. Vital Signs

Vital signs are the most basic and critical indicators of a patient's health. They provide real-time data on the patient's cardiovascular and respiratory systems, offering key insights into any changes in their condition. Regular monitoring and documentation of vital signs are essential to tracking patient progress and identifying potential issues.

Example:

BP: 135/80 mmHg, HR: 82 bpm, RR: 18 breaths/min, Temp: 36.9°C, SpO2: 97% on room air at 8:00 AM.

Abnormal vital signs should trigger further assessments or interventions, and these actions must be recorded as well. For instance, if the patient's blood pressure rises significantly, you must document the follow-up, such as notifying the physician and administering medication.

2. Medications

Medication administration is another critical area of nursing documentation. Medications are often one of the primary ways patient care is managed, and errors in this area can lead to serious complications. Proper documentation should include the name of the medication, dosage, route of administration, time given, and patient response.

Example:

Administered 5 mg Morphine IV at 10:00 AM for pain rated at 8/10. Patient reported pain decreased to 4/10 at 10:30 AM.

In addition to regularly scheduled medications, it's equally important to document any PRN (as-needed) medications, especially in cases where pain management is a central concern. If a patient requests additional medication outside of the regular schedule, be sure to note the reason for the request, the dose given, and the patient's response.

3. Interventions and Procedures

Nursing interventions, such as administering IV fluids, inserting a catheter, or performing wound care, must be documented with specific detail. Each intervention should include the type of procedure, time performed, technique used, and the patient's response to the intervention.

Example:

Inserted Foley catheter using sterile technique at 10:30 AM. 350 mL of clear yellow urine drained immediately. Patient tolerated the procedure without discomfort.

Documentation of interventions ensures that all members of the healthcare team are aware of the care provided, while also serving as legal evidence that appropriate procedures were followed.

4. Patient Reactions and Outcomes

After administering treatments or performing procedures, it's essential to record the patient's response. How the patient reacts to care, including any adverse reactions, should be meticulously noted.

Example:

Patient experienced mild nausea 15 minutes after administration of 100 mg Vancomycin IV. Reported symptoms to attending physician, who prescribed anti-nausea medication.

Capturing patient reactions is not just important for tracking progress, but also for identifying any potential complications. Documenting the patient's outcome after interventions—whether it's a medication or physical therapy—provides a clear timeline of their response to treatment.

5. Communication with the Healthcare Team

Nursing is a collaborative practice, and clear communication with physicians, specialists, and other nurses is essential to ensuring that patients receive coordinated, effective care. Any significant changes in the patient's condition should be communicated to the appropriate team members, and these conversations should be documented in the patient's record.

Example:

Notified Dr. Jones at 12:00 PM of patient's persistent tachycardia (HR 110 bpm) despite administration of beta-blocker. New order received for additional cardiac monitoring.

This documentation ensures that there is a clear trail of communication and that the healthcare team is working with up-to-date information, reducing the risk of errors or misunderstandings.

6. Patient Education

Educating patients about their treatment and care is a critical component of nursing. Proper documentation of education ensures that patients are well-informed about managing their condition, taking medications, and recognizing warning signs.

Example:

Educated patient on proper wound care at 3:00 PM. Demonstrated cleaning and dressing change technique. Patient verbalized understanding and performed the task with supervision.

Documenting patient education also provides legal protection by showing that the patient was properly informed and involved in their care.

What to Avoid: Over-Documentation vs. Under-Documentation

While thorough documentation is essential, both over-documentation and under-documentation can lead to problems. Let's explore the balance required in documentation practices.

Over-Documentation

Over-documentation occurs when nurses include irrelevant details or an excessive amount of information that does not contribute to the overall understanding of the patient's care. This can obscure important clinical details and create confusion for other members of the healthcare team.

Example of Over-Documentation:

"Patient woke up at 7:00 AM, asked for water at 7:15 AM, drank half a glass of water, watched TV for 10 minutes, and then requested a blanket at 7:30 AM."

While these details may be accurate, they are not relevant to the clinical care being provided. Over-documentation clutters the record, making it harder for healthcare providers to quickly identify important information.

Under-Documentation

On the other hand, under-documentation can have more serious legal and clinical implications. Failing to include key details or leaving gaps in the record can imply that care was not provided, even if it was. If a nurse does not document an intervention, for instance, it may appear as though the patient's needs were neglected.

Example of Under-Documentation:

"Patient received medication. Vital signs stable."

This vague note leaves out critical information, such as what medication was given, at what dose, and how the patient responded. In the event of an audit or legal investigation, under-documentation like this could be used to argue that care was inadequate or incomplete.

Legal Ramifications of Documentation Errors

The way nurses document patient care can have significant legal implications, particularly if the care provided is ever questioned in court or during a disciplinary review. Both over- and under-documentation can lead to legal risks.

Legal Risks of Over-Documentation

Over-documentation can result in contradictions within the patient's record, which could be used against you in legal cases. For example, if you provide an excessive level of detail about a patient's behavior but fail to note important clinical data, a lawyer could argue that you were focused on irrelevant details rather than essential care.

Legal Risks of Under-Documentation

Under-documentation poses an even greater legal risk. If an important detail is missing from the record—such as the administration of medication or a significant change in the patient's condition—it can be assumed that the action was not taken. In the eyes of the law, if it wasn't documented, it didn't happen. This could lead to accusations of negligence or malpractice, even if the nurse provided the appropriate care.

For example, in a case where a nurse failed to document the administration of a life-saving medication during a patient's critical decline, the lack of documentation was used as evidence in a lawsuit, leading to significant legal consequences for the nurse and the hospital.

Daily nursing documentation is one of the most critical aspects of ensuring quality patient care and legal protection. The essential components of nursing records—such as vital signs, medications, patient reactions, interventions, communication, and education—must be meticulously documented. At the same time, striking a balance is crucial: avoid over-documentation, which can cloud the record with irrelevant details, and steer clear of under-documentation, which can leave dangerous gaps in the care narrative. By mastering these documentation practices, you protect both your patients and your professional license.

CHAPTER 5

Charting in High-Stress Situations: Emergencies and Critical Care

In the world of nursing, high-stress environments like emergency rooms (ERs) and critical care units (ICUs) are fast-paced, chaotic, and often overwhelming. In these situations, nurses must make quick, life-saving decisions while simultaneously documenting critical interventions. Maintaining accurate, clear, and thorough documentation under these conditions is a challenge but is essential for patient safety, continuity of care, and legal protection.

Nurses are often under immense pressure to stabilize patients quickly while juggling various tasks: administering medications, performing procedures, and communicating with physicians and family members. In the midst of this whirlwind, documentation can sometimes be seen as secondary. However, the consequences of poor documentation in high-pressure situations can be severe. This chapter delves into the strategies for prioritizing documentation during chaotic moments and why detailed charting in emergencies is crucial for both legal protection and patient safety.

Why Detailed Documentation Is Crucial in Emergencies

Emergency and critical care environments demand quick decision-making and immediate actions. In these situations, comprehensive documentation is vital for several reasons:

Legal Protection: In emergency situations, the outcomes are often unpredictable. If a patient's condition worsens, leading to negative outcomes such as permanent injury or death, detailed documentation provides a clear record of the care provided. This documentation is essential if the nurse's actions are later questioned in a legal setting. Without proper records, it can be difficult to prove that the correct care was provided in a timely manner.

Example: Imagine a situation where a trauma patient arrives in the ER after a severe car accident. The nursing team initiates CPR, administers emergency medications, and calls for the on-duty physician. Unfortunately, despite all efforts, the patient dies. In the aftermath, the family files a lawsuit claiming negligence, suggesting that the care provided was insufficient. Here, the detailed records of every intervention—timing of medication, duration of CPR, and communication with the physician—can serve as proof that the nursing team followed protocol and did everything within their capacity to save the patient. Without these records, the nurse may face scrutiny and potential legal consequences.

Continuity of Care: In emergencies, many healthcare providers often work on the same patient across different shifts or departments. Accurate and up-to-date charting ensures that each team knows exactly what interventions have been performed and how the patient has responded. This continuity of care is crucial for avoiding redundant treatments or missing essential steps in the patient's care plan.

Example: A patient in cardiac arrest is transferred from the ER to the ICU after initial resuscitation. The ICU team relies heavily on the ER notes to understand what medications were given, what dosages were used, how the patient responded, and what interventions are still needed. If these details are not clearly documented, it can lead to repeated treatments or missed steps in the patient's care, which could negatively impact their recovery.

Patient Safety: In high-stress situations, detailed documentation helps protect patients by providing a clear timeline of events. Proper charting ensures that each team member knows what care has been provided, preventing errors such as missed doses of medication or the failure to monitor vital signs. These records are essential for making informed clinical decisions in real time.

Example: Imagine a patient arrives in critical condition, and the nurse documents administering a high-risk medication, such as epinephrine. Later, if the patient's condition deteriorates, the medical team will rely on the documentation to determine whether additional doses of epinephrine are needed or whether the patient is having an adverse reaction to a different intervention. Without proper documentation, there could be confusion about whether medication was given, leading to either under- or over-treatment.

Strategies for Prioritizing Documentation in High-Stress Situations

Maintaining proper documentation in high-stress environments requires nurses to prioritize what to document first, ensure accuracy despite time pressures, and use strategies to streamline the process without sacrificing detail.

1. Prioritize Critical Interventions and Vital Signs

In the chaos of an emergency, not everything can be documented in real-time. Therefore, prioritization is key. Focus on documenting the most critical interventions and vital signs as soon as possible. This includes noting:

Time of emergency onset: It's important to establish a clear timeline of when the situation began. For example, "Patient found unresponsive at 12:10 PM" sets the stage for everything that follows.

Initial vital signs and subsequent changes: Documenting key vital signs such as heart rate, blood pressure, oxygen saturation, and respiratory rate at regular intervals provides a critical overview of the patient's status. Vital sign trends during an emergency help guide treatment decisions.

Critical interventions: Any life-saving interventions—like CPR, defibrillation, intubation, or the administration of medications like epinephrine or vasopressors—should be recorded with precise timing. For example, "CPR initiated at 12:12 PM, first defibrillation shock delivered at 12:14 PM" provides a clear and concise record of interventions.

Example: In a code situation, the nurse in charge of documentation should immediately record when CPR is started, when medications such as epinephrine are administered, and any significant changes in the patient's condition. These are the key interventions that must be documented in real-time to ensure an accurate account of the care provided.

2. Document the Patient's Response to Interventions

It's not enough to simply record what interventions were performed—how the patient responded to those interventions is equally important. Documenting whether the patient's condition improved, deteriorated, or remained stable helps guide subsequent treatment.

Example: After administering epinephrine during cardiac arrest, the nurse might write, "Patient's heart rate increased to 80 bpm at 12:16 PM after administration of 1 mg epinephrine IV. Spontaneous circulation restored at 12:18 PM." This provides a clear cause-and-effect record of the patient's response.

This information is crucial, as it demonstrates that the care provided had a measurable impact and helps to justify continued or altered treatment approaches.

3. Leverage Teamwork for Documentation

In critical care environments, it's common for multiple nurses and healthcare professionals to work on a patient simultaneously. Using teamwork to divide tasks can ensure that documentation is completed without compromising patient care.

Example: During a resuscitation attempt, one nurse might take responsibility for documenting events while the other nurses focus on hands-on patient care. The nurse documenting can quickly note the time of medication administration, interventions like intubation, and any changes in the patient's condition. This division of labor allows for both rapid intervention and accurate documentation.

4. Use Approved Abbreviations and Shortcuts

When time is of the essence, using approved medical abbreviations and shortcuts can help streamline documentation while maintaining accuracy. However, it's essential to ensure that all abbreviations are universally understood within your facility to avoid confusion later.

Example: Rather than writing out "Cardiopulmonary resuscitation," the nurse can simply document "CPR initiated at 12:12 PM." Similarly, using "SOB" for shortness of breath or "IV" for intravenous can save time without sacrificing clarity.

Using shorthand in emergencies helps speed up the documentation process, but it's important to balance this with ensuring that the record remains clear and understandable for all healthcare providers.

5. Jot Down Key Times and Events for Later Entry

In particularly chaotic situations, it might be impossible to document everything in real-time. In these cases, quickly jotting down key times and events on paper or a whiteboard can help capture the necessary information for later entry into the patient's chart.

Example: During a major trauma, a nurse might keep a quick log of when medications were administered or when procedures like intubation occurred. Once the situation is under control, these notes can be entered into the chart with more detailed descriptions.

This strategy ensures that no critical information is lost, even if the nurse is unable to chart immediately. However, it's important to ensure that the notes are transcribed into the official record as soon as possible to maintain accuracy.

Avoiding Common Pitfalls in Emergency Documentation

Despite the chaos of emergencies, it's important to avoid some common documentation pitfalls that can lead to legal or clinical complications later.

1. Avoid Delayed Charting

While it's understandable that emergencies might delay documentation, waiting too long to document can lead to inaccuracies or missing information. The longer the delay, the more likely it is that critical details will be forgotten, leading to gaps in the care record.

Legal Ramification: In a case where documentation was delayed for hours after a critical event, the nurse was unable to recall the exact timing of interventions. In court, this lack of real-time documentation was used to argue that the care provided was substandard, leading to a costly legal settlement.

2. Be Objective, Not Subjective

Even in high-stress situations, it's important to keep documentation objective and free of personal opinion. Avoid phrases like "patient seemed anxious" and instead describe what you observed. For example, "Patient was pacing, sweating, and reported chest pain" provides clear, factual observations without introducing subjectivity.

Example: Instead of writing "patient appeared scared," document, "Patient was shaking, with widened eyes, and verbally expressed fear of intubation." This kind of objective documentation is crucial for providing a clear, unbiased account of the patient's condition.

In high-stress environments like emergencies and critical care, accurate and timely documentation is not just a professional obligation—it is a critical tool for ensuring patient safety, continuity of care, and legal protection. By prioritizing essential details like vital signs, critical interventions, and patient responses, nurses can provide clear, concise recordsIn high-stress environments like emergency rooms and critical care, accurate and timely documentation is not just a professional obligation—it is a critical tool for ensuring patient safety, continuity of care, and legal protection. By prioritizing essential details like vital signs, critical interventions, and patient responses, nurses can provide clear, concise records that protect their patients and themselves.

Accurate charting prevents errors, helps other team members respond appropriately, and serves as a solid legal record should a situation be called into question. As nurses navigate these chaotic moments, using efficient documentation strategies, such as abbreviations and teamwork, will ensure that patient care remains the priority without compromising the legal and professional requirements for documentation.

CHAPTER 6

Electronic Health Records (EHR): Navigating Modern Charting Tools

The healthcare industry's shift from paper charts to Electronic Health Records (EHRs) has significantly transformed the way patient care is documented. EHRs provide a comprehensive, real-time overview of a patient's medical history and treatment, improving access to vital data and promoting better care coordination across healthcare teams. However, as with any technological advancement, this transition comes with challenges. For nurses, mastering EHR systems is essential to providing accurate, efficient care while avoiding the common pitfalls that can lead to errors or missed information.

In this chapter, we will explore the benefits of EHRs over traditional paper charts, provide tips for maximizing efficiency and accuracy with EHR systems, and highlight common mistakes that nurses should avoid to ensure the best patient outcomes and legal protection.

The Transition from Paper Charts to EHRs

The transition from paper-based charting to EHRs has been one of the most significant changes in healthcare over the past few decades. While paper charts have served nurses for generations, they present numerous challenges, such as illegible handwriting, difficulty in sharing information between departments, and the risk of physical damage or loss. EHRs have addressed many of these issues and have brought about improvements in the way patient care is documented and managed.

Advantages of EHRs Over Paper Charts

Legibility and Standardization: One of the most immediate advantages of EHRs is that they eliminate the issue of illegible handwriting.

Standardized digital entries ensure that all information is clear and readable, which reduces the risk of misinterpretation and improves communication between healthcare providers. This is particularly crucial in fast-paced environments like emergency rooms where quick, accurate decisions can save lives.

Real-Time Updates: Unlike paper charts, which can be delayed by the need to physically retrieve and update documents, EHRs allow for real-time updates. When a patient's status changes—whether it's a lab result, a new medication order, or a vital sign—the information is instantly available to all members of the healthcare team. This real-time access enhances decision-making and allows for immediate interventions when needed.

Improved Data Integration: EHRs provide a centralized platform where all aspects of a patient's care are integrated. This includes not only nursing notes but also lab results, radiology reports, medication histories, and treatment plans. Having all this information in one place enables healthcare providers to make more informed decisions and reduces the risk of fragmented or incomplete care.

Enhanced Communication: EHRs improve communication across various departments and healthcare providers. When a patient is transferred from the emergency room to the ICU or discharged to a long-term care facility, the receiving team can access the patient's complete medical history, ensuring continuity of care.

Increased Security and Compliance: EHR systems are equipped with security measures such as encryption and access controls, which protect patient data from unauthorized access. Additionally, EHRs ensure compliance with regulations like HIPAA by automatically tracking who accesses patient records and when. This reduces the risk of privacy violations and ensures that sensitive information is handled appropriately.

Challenges of the Transition

While EHRs offer numerous benefits, the transition from paper charts has not been without its challenges, particularly for nurses who are accustomed to paper-based systems. Some of the main challenges include:

Steep Learning Curve: EHR systems vary in complexity, and some nurses—especially those who have been practicing for many years—may find it difficult to adapt to the new technology. The interface of EHR systems can be overwhelming, particularly for those unfamiliar with digital systems.

Time-Consuming Data Entry: EHRs often require more detailed data entry than paper charts, leading to documentation fatigue. Nurses may feel that they are spending too much time in front of a computer and not enough time interacting with their patients. This can lead to frustration and decreased job satisfaction

Over-Reliance on Templates: Many EHR systems use templated notes, which can streamline documentation but also encourage nurses to rely on auto-populated fields that may not fully capture a patient's unique condition. This over-reliance on templates can lead to generic or incomplete records, ultimately affecting patient care.

Tips for Maximizing Accuracy and Efficiency with EHRs

Mastering EHRs requires a combination of technical proficiency, critical thinking, and attention to detail. Here are some strategies that can help nurses make the most of their EHR systems:

1. Understand the System Thoroughly

Becoming familiar with your EHR system's interface is the first step toward efficient charting. Take advantage of any training sessions offered by your healthcare facility, and don't hesitate to seek out additional resources like online tutorials or user guides. Understanding the nuances of your system will help you navigate it more efficiently during your shift.

Tip: Spend time familiarizing yourself with the layout of the system when you're not under pressure. Practice accessing critical areas like medication administration records, lab results, and patient assessments so that you can find them quickly when needed. Some systems also allow for customization, so take the time to arrange your workspace to fit your workflow.

2. Use Templates Wisely, But Customize Entries

Many EHR systems provide templates for common nursing tasks, such as recording vital signs or administering medications. While these templates can save time, it's important to customize them to reflect the patient's actual condition and responses. Avoid simply clicking through pre-populated fields without reviewing them carefully.

Tip: If a template auto-populates "normal" values for vital signs, ensure that you manually update the fields with the patient's actual readings. For example, if a patient's blood pressure is elevated or their oxygen saturation is low, make sure these values are documented accurately instead of leaving the default normal values.

3. Double-Check Critical Entries

EHRs allow for rapid data entry, but this speed can also lead to errors if entries are not carefully reviewed. Incorrect medication entries, wrong dosages, or inaccurate times can have serious consequences for the patient's care.

Tip: Always double-check critical entries such as medication orders, dosages, patient allergies, and the patient's identifying information. EHRs often have built-in safety features like alerts for potential drug interactions or allergies, but these systems are not infallible. Developing the habit of reviewing your entries before finalizing them can prevent costly mistakes.

4. Document in Real-Time When Possible

Real-time documentation is one of the greatest advantages of EHRs, but it can be challenging to maintain during busy shifts. Whenever possible, try to document care as it happens rather than relying on memory to fill in details later. Real-time documentation ensures that your notes are accurate and reduces the likelihood of missing key information.

Tip: If you can't document in real-time, jot down quick notes on a notepad or in your phone (if allowed) to capture important events. For example, if you administered pain medication or performed a dressing change, write down the time and details so you can enter them into the EHR later without missing anything.

5. Use System Alerts and Reminders

Many EHR systems come with built-in reminders for tasks such as medication administration or patient assessments. These alerts can help ensure that nothing falls through the cracks during a busy shift. Make use of these tools to stay on top of your patient care tasks.

Tip: Set reminders for tasks that must be performed at specific intervals, such as rechecking a patient's blood sugar levels after administering insulin or reassessing a patient's pain level after administering medication.

Common EHR Mistakes and How to Avoid Them

Despite the many advantages of EHRs, there are common mistakes that nurses must be mindful of to avoid compromising patient safety and care.

1. Over-reliance on Auto-Population

Auto-population features are designed to save time, but they can lead to significant errors if not carefully reviewed. For example, copying and pasting notes from a previous shift without updating them can result in outdated or inaccurate information.

Example: A nurse copies a note from a previous shift that reads, "Patient reports no pain," even though during the current shift, the patient is experiencing severe pain. This mistake can lead to inappropriate pain management and a negative outcome for the patient.

Solution: Always review and update auto-populated fields or copied notes to ensure that they reflect the patient's current condition. Avoid relying solely on previous documentation, even if it appears to be accurate.

2. Click Fatigue and Documentation Overload

EHRs often require nurses to navigate through multiple windows, tabs, and checkboxes to document patient care. This can lead to "click fatigue," where nurses become overwhelmed by the sheer number of clicks needed to complete a task. In turn, this can lead to errors or incomplete documentation.

Solution: Customize your EHR interface to streamline your workflow. Many systems allow users to arrange frequently used tabs in a way that minimizes the number of clicks required to document care. Additionally, learn the shortcuts specific to your system to speed up navigation.

3. Failure to Document Communication with Other Healthcare Providers

In fast-paced healthcare environments, nurses often communicate directly with physicians, pharmacists, or other team members about patient care decisions. Failing to document these conversations can lead to gaps in the patient's record, making it difficult for others to understand the rationale behind certain decisions.

Example: A nurse communicates with the attending physician about a patient's adverse reaction to a medication. The physician provides new orders, but the nurse fails to document the conversation or the changes in the care plan. Later, another nurse or physician may be unaware of the updated orders, leading to potential harm.

Solution: Document every significant communication with other healthcare providers, including the time,###

Chapter 7

Protecting Your License: Documenting Incidents, Errors, and Near Misses

As a nurse, your professional license is your most valuable asset, and protecting it requires a thorough understanding of how to document incidents, medication errors, and near misses. Proper documentation in these situations serves not only to ensure patient safety but also to provide legal protection for the nurse and the healthcare facility. In this chapter, we will explore the best practices for documenting incidents, errors, and near misses, the role of incident reports, the legal implications of improper documentation, and how to balance transparency with professional judgment.

The Importance of Proper Documentation in Incidents, Errors, and Near Misses

Healthcare is a high-stakes field where the unexpected can occur. Even the most experienced nurses may encounter situations where an error or near miss happens. These can range from medication errors to patient falls, and they must be documented with the same level of care as any other aspect of patient care.

Proper documentation of these events is essential for several reasons:

1. **Ensuring Patient Safety**: Documenting incidents and near misses can help prevent future errors by highlighting areas that need improvement. For example, documenting a near miss involving medication can lead to adjustments in the workflow or identification of system flaws.

2. **Protecting Your License**: Errors and incidents, if not properly documented, can lead to legal scrutiny. Accurate,

transparent documentation shows that you have acted responsibly and appropriately, even when things go wrong. It can be your strongest defense if legal actions are taken against you.

3. **Legal Requirements**: Many state nursing boards and healthcare facilities have strict requirements for documenting errors and adverse events. Failing to comply with these standards could result in disciplinary actions, including fines or loss of licensure.

Example:

Consider a nurse who administers the wrong dosage of insulin to a patient. The error is recognized before causing harm, but instead of documenting the mistake, the nurse decides not to report it, fearing repercussions. Later, when the patient experiences hypoglycemia, the error comes to light. Because it was not documented, the nurse's failure to report the incident may be viewed as negligence, which could lead to disciplinary action or even legal consequences.

How to Properly Chart Incidents, Medication Errors, and Adverse Events

When documenting incidents, errors, or near misses, the key is to maintain clarity, accuracy, and objectivity. Here are best practices to follow:

1. Stick to the Facts

When documenting an error or incident, it is critical to include factual, objective information. Avoid assigning blame or speculating about causes. Instead, focus on what happened, when it happened, and how it was addressed.

- **Example**: Instead of writing, "The nurse gave the wrong medication due to being overwhelmed," write, "Administered 5 mg of Hydromorphone IV at 10:00 AM. Correct order was for 0.5 mg Hydromorphone IV. Notified physician immediately."

This entry provides a clear, factual account of what occurred without suggesting personal opinions or assumptions about the nurse's emotional state or reasons for the error.

2. Include Relevant Details

For every incident or error, provide as many relevant details as possible. These might include:

- **Time and date of the event.**

- **Actions taken immediately following the incident,** such as notifying the physician, contacting the charge nurse, or monitoring the patient for adverse effects.

- **Patient's response or reaction,** such as changes in vital signs or reported symptoms.

- **Any corrective actions taken,** such as administering a reversal agent or discontinuing a treatment.

- **Example**: "At 10:05 AM, after administering incorrect medication, patient's BP decreased to 90/60. Notified Dr. Smith at 10:10 AM. Order received to monitor BP every 15 minutes for the next hour and administer IV fluids."

3. Document Patient Notifications

In many cases, patients or their families need to be informed of an error or adverse event. This is a sensitive but important aspect of transparent care. It is crucial to document when and how the patient or their family was informed.

- **Example**: "At 10:15 AM, patient informed of the medication error. Explained monitoring plan for the next hour and answered patient's questions regarding potential side effects."

4. Follow Facility Policies

Every healthcare facility will have its own policies for documenting incidents and errors, as well as a system for filing incident reports (discussed in the next section). Familiarize yourself with your facility's procedures to ensure compliance with institutional standards. Some facilities may have specific templates or forms that must be used.

- **Tip:** Always document within the patient's medical record any interventions or assessments following an error. However, internal reports (incident reports) should not be included in the medical record, as they are separate and intended for risk management.

The Role of Incident Reports and Legal Implications

In addition to documenting the event in the patient's medical record, most healthcare institutions require that an **incident report** be filed when an error or near miss occurs. Incident reports are crucial for tracking safety concerns, identifying patterns, and making system-wide improvements. These reports also have significant legal implications, so it's important to understand their role and how to use them effectively.

1. What Is an Incident Report?

An incident report is a formal document used to record details about an adverse event, error, or near miss that occurred within the healthcare facility. These reports are typically not part of the patient's medical record and are used internally to review and improve safety procedures.

- **Example of incidents requiring a report:**
    - Medication errors (wrong drug, wrong dose, or wrong route).
    - Patient falls.

- o   Needle stick injuries.
- o   Equipment malfunctions that affected patient care.
- o   Miscommunication between team members that leads to an error.

2. How to File an Incident Report

When completing an incident report, it is important to provide a factual, non-judgmental account of the event. Similar to charting in the medical record, incident reports should include the following:

- **Who was involved** (patient name, healthcare providers).
- **What occurred** (specifics of the incident or error).
- **Where and when it happened** (location and time).
- **Why and how it occurred**, if known.
- **Actions taken to mitigate the situation.**
- **Example**: A nurse files an incident report after discovering that a patient was given medication intended for another patient. The report includes the time, details of the medication mix-up, the physician's notification, and the actions taken to monitor and stabilize the patient.

3. Legal Implications of Incident Reports

Incident reports play a critical role in **risk management** and **legal protection** for healthcare providers and facilities. These reports are generally not discoverable in court, meaning they are used internally and not part of legal proceedings. However, failure to file an incident report or filing a report with inaccuracies can have serious legal consequences.

- **Example**: If a patient experiences harm due to a medication error and no incident report is filed, the nurse and the healthcare facility could be held liable for failing to address a safety issue. In contrast, filing a detailed incident report shows that the healthcare team took immediate steps to manage the error and prevent future occurrences.

Balancing Transparency with Professional Judgment

Documenting errors and adverse events requires transparency, but it also demands careful judgment. You must be honest and thorough while also protecting patient confidentiality and adhering to legal standards. Here are a few principles to follow:

1. Be Transparent but Objective

Honesty is key in documenting errors, but avoid unnecessary details or emotional language that could cast the event in a negative light. Stick to the facts and avoid speculating about fault or intent.

- **Example**: Instead of writing, "I accidentally gave the wrong medication because I was distracted," document, "Administered 100 mg of XYZ medication at 9:00 AM, intended dose was 10 mg. Immediately notified physician, and corrective action taken."

2. Do Not Include Incident Reports in the Patient's Medical Record

As mentioned earlier, incident reports are separate from the medical record. Avoid referencing the existence of an incident report in the patient's chart, as this could make the report accessible during legal proceedings.

- **Example**: Do not write, "An incident report was filed for this event" in the patient's record. Simply document the facts of the incident and the actions taken to address it.

3. Maintain Patient Confidentiality

When documenting an error that involves another patient (e.g., a medication intended for one patient is given to another), ensure that you maintain confidentiality. Do not include identifying information about the other patient involved in the error.

- **Example**: Instead of writing, "Medication intended for Mr. A was given to Mr. B," document the event without using the other patient's name: "Medication intended for another patient was administered to Mr. B in error."

Documenting incidents, errors, and near misses is a critical aspect of nursing practice that serves to protect both patient safety and your nursing license. By adhering to best practices—such as sticking to facts, following facility policies, and using incident reports properly—you can ensure that your documentation is clear, accurate, and legally sound. Balancing transparency with professional judgment is key to maintaining both patient trust and legal protection. In the next chapter, we'll explore how to prepare your documentation for audits and investigations, ensuring that your records are comprehensive and compliant with regulatory standards.

Chapter 8

Audit-Proofing Your Documentation: Preparing for Investigations

Nursing documentation serves multiple purposes—facilitating patient care, ensuring continuity among healthcare teams, and providing a legal record of the care delivered. However, it also plays a critical role in audits and investigations, where every entry may be scrutinized for accuracy, completeness, and compliance with healthcare regulations. Audit-proofing your documentation is essential to safeguard both your nursing license and the facility you work for. In this chapter, we'll dive into how nursing records are used in audits, how to ensure that your charts stand up to scrutiny, and strategies to maintain consistent and compliant documentation.

The Role of Nursing Records in Audits and Investigations

In healthcare, audits and investigations can be initiated for various reasons, such as routine compliance checks, internal quality control reviews, or external investigations related to legal disputes or insurance claims. In these situations, nursing records are often one of the primary sources of information used to assess whether the appropriate standards of care were met.

1. Routine Audits

Healthcare organizations frequently conduct routine audits to ensure that documentation meets both internal standards and external regulatory requirements (such as those from the Joint Commission or Centers for Medicare & Medicaid Services, CMS). These audits typically review patient records to verify that care was documented correctly and that all necessary elements (e.g., assessments, medication administration, and patient education) were completed in accordance with protocols.

Example: A facility conducting a CMS compliance audit might review patient charts to verify that all assessments were performed at the required intervals and that pain management interventions were properly documented.

2. Investigations Following an Adverse Event

When an adverse event occurs, such as a patient injury or medication error, an investigation may follow to determine the cause and whether negligence was involved. Nursing records serve as the official account of the care provided and will be scrutinized for consistency, completeness, and accuracy.

Example: In the case of a patient fall, an investigation would look at the documentation for details about the patient's condition before and after the fall, any safety precautions taken, and whether the incident was documented according to facility protocols.

3. Insurance and Legal Investigations

In cases where claims or lawsuits are filed, patient records become legal documents. Attorneys, insurance companies, and sometimes even courts will review nursing documentation to determine whether the care provided met the standard of care and whether there was any deviation that contributed to the patient's harm.

Example: If a patient suffers an adverse reaction to a medication and later files a lawsuit, the patient's medical records will be examined to ensure that the correct dosage and route of administration were documented, along with any follow-up care provided after the reaction.

Ensuring Your Charts Stand Up to Scrutiny

When your documentation is under audit or investigation, it is essential that it can withstand rigorous scrutiny. Below are key elements that auditors and investigators will look for in nursing documentation, and strategies for ensuring that your charts are bulletproof.

1. Consistency

Inconsistent documentation raises red flags for auditors and investigators. Entries must be aligned with each other across different parts of the patient's record, including physician orders, nursing notes, and medication administration records. Any discrepancies between these sections can suggest incomplete care or even falsification of records.

Example: Suppose a patient's chart notes that pain medication was given at 3:00 PM, but the nurse's narrative documentation does not mention assessing the patient's pain level before or after administration. This inconsistency could be seen as a lack of proper pain management and would likely be flagged during an audit.

Strategy:

Always ensure that related entries (e.g., assessments and interventions) are consistent with each other across the patient's record.

For medication administration, document both the administration itself and the patient's response, ensuring the timeline makes sense.

2. Accuracy

Accurate documentation is essential, particularly when it comes to vital signs, medication administration, and patient assessments. Even small inaccuracies—such as recording the wrong time of an intervention—can have significant legal and clinical consequences.

Example: If a nurse administers a critical medication at 10:00 AM but documents it as being given at 9:00 AM, this discrepancy can cause confusion about whether the patient received the correct treatment at the right time.

Strategy:

Double-check entries before finalizing them, especially those related to vital signs, medication dosages, and times.

Use the EHR's time-stamping function to record real-time actions, ensuring that your documentation reflects what occurred.

3. Completeness

Incomplete documentation is one of the most common issues found during audits. If key elements of patient care are missing from the chart—such as failure to document an assessment, intervention, or follow-up—it can appear as though those actions were never performed.

Example: A nurse assesses a patient after surgery but fails to document checking for signs of infection. Later, if the patient develops an infection, the absence of documentation could be interpreted as negligence or failure to provide appropriate post-operative care.

Strategy:

Use structured formats like SOAP (Subjective, Objective, Assessment, Plan) or DAR (Data, Action, Response) to ensure that your documentation is complete.

Always include follow-up care, particularly after interventions like pain management, wound care, or medication administration.

4. Timeliness

Timely documentation is critical, especially when it comes to audits. Documenting events in real-time (or as close to real-time as possible) ensures that records are accurate and that the timeline of patient care is clear.

Example: In a patient experiencing cardiac arrest, if life-saving interventions are documented hours after they occurred, this delay could cast doubt on whether the interventions were provided in a timely manner, affecting both clinical and legal evaluations.

Strategy:

Prioritize real-time documentation whenever possible, and avoid retrospective charting unless absolutely necessary. If you must document after the fact, clearly state that the entry is a "late entry" and explain the reason for the delay.

Strategies for Maintaining Consistent and Compliant Documentation

Audit-proofing your documentation isn't just about addressing errors retroactively. The best approach is to adopt strategies that ensure your charts are consistent and compliant from the start. Below are some strategies to help maintain high-quality documentation.

1. Use Structured Documentation Formats

Using structured formats such as SOAP (Subjective, Objective, Assessment, Plan) or DAR (Data, Action, Response) helps ensure that your documentation is both comprehensive and organized. Structured formats guide you through the essential components of each entry, helping to prevent omissions and ensuring that key details are not overlooked.

SOAP Example:

Subjective: Patient reports 8/10 pain in the left leg.

Objective: BP 130/80, HR 78, no swelling or redness in the left leg.

Assessment: Possible post-operative pain; no signs of infection.

Plan: Administer 5 mg morphine IV as ordered, recheck pain level in 30 minutes.

2. Consistency Across the Care Team

Consistency in documentation is critical when multiple healthcare providers are involved in a patient's care. Nurses, physicians, and other members of the care team must ensure that their notes align and that there are no discrepancies in the chart.

Strategy:

Communicate regularly with other members of the healthcare team about the patient's condition and ensure that changes to the care plan are documented accurately by all providers.

Cross-reference your documentation with physician orders and progress notes to ensure consistency.

3. Avoid "Charting by Exception" Unless Appropriate

"Charting by exception" means documenting only deviations from normal findings. While this can save time, it can also lead to incomplete records if used inappropriately. Auditors may question whether full assessments were performed if routine observations are not charted.

Example: If you fail to document normal vital signs and instead only document when they become abnormal, it may appear that routine checks were missed.

Strategy:

Use charting by exception only when permitted by facility policy and ensure that even normal findings are recorded when necessary, especially for high-risk patients or in critical situations.

4. Incorporate Checklists into Your Workflow

Checklists are a valuable tool for ensuring that no steps are missed during patient care, and they can also serve as a reference for your documentation. Many EHR systems allow nurses to use built-in checklists to guide their documentation of routine tasks.

Strategy:

Utilize checklists to prompt assessments, interventions, and follow-ups. For example, use a checklist when administering a complex medication regimen to ensure that each step—such as checking allergies and documenting patient responses—is recorded.

5. Anticipate Audits and Be Proactive

Rather than viewing audits as a reactive process, anticipate that your documentation may be reviewed at any time. This mindset ensures that your records are always audit-ready, reducing the likelihood of errors or omissions.

Strategy:

Review your own documentation regularly, especially for high-risk patients or complex cases.

Attend training sessions on documentation best practices and audit preparation to stay updated on compliance standards.

Audit-proofing your nursing documentation is essential to protecting your professional license, ensuring patient safety, and maintaining legal compliance. By understanding how your charts are used in audits and investigations, and by adopting strategies to ensure consistency, accuracy, completeness, and timeliness, you can create records that stand up to scrutiny. Structured documentation, consistent care-team communication, and a proactive approach to documentation compliance will not only protect you during audits but also ensure the highest standard of care for your patients.

Chapter 9

Defensive Documentation: Protecting Yourself in Litigation

In the world of healthcare, providing excellent patient care is always the top priority. However, in an increasingly litigious society, nurses must also be vigilant about how they document that care. Defensive documentation refers to maintaining comprehensive, accurate, and timely records that not only support patient care but also protect you legally in case of lawsuits or investigations. Every entry in a patient's chart can become a piece of evidence, and the quality of that documentation can either support or undermine your defense if a legal challenge arises.

In this chapter, we'll explore how nursing documentation is used in litigation, charting practices that can protect you in court, and how to respond if your documentation is called into question.

How Nursing Documentation is Used in Lawsuits

In any healthcare-related lawsuit, whether it involves malpractice, negligence, or wrongful death, nursing documentation serves as a key piece of evidence. The goal of litigation is often to determine whether the standard of care was followed, and nursing notes provide a detailed account of how care was provided, what interventions were performed, and how the patient responded.

1. Medical Malpractice Claims

In medical malpractice cases, the plaintiff (typically the patient or their family) must prove that:

The nurse had a duty of care to the patient.

The nurse breached this duty by failing to meet the standard of care.

This breach of duty directly caused harm to the patient (causation).

The patient suffered damages (physical, financial, or emotional) as a result.

Nursing documentation is key to defending against these claims. If your documentation is detailed, accurate, and consistent, it can demonstrate that you fulfilled your duty of care and met the standard of care expected in that situation. If your documentation is incomplete, inaccurate, or inconsistent, it may be used to support the claim that care was substandard.

Example: If a patient experiences complications after surgery and claims that post-operative care was inadequate, your documentation can provide evidence of the care you provided. If you documented wound assessments, patient education on infection risks, and timely communication with the physician about any concerns, these entries can show that you acted in accordance with nursing standards.

2. Negligence Cases

In cases of negligence, nursing documentation may be scrutinized to determine if the nurse failed to act appropriately in response to a patient's condition. This could involve failing to monitor a patient adequately, not reporting significant changes to the physician, or failing to follow established protocols.

Example: A patient who suffers a fall while in the hospital may file a lawsuit claiming that the nursing staff failed to take appropriate fall precautions. If your documentation shows that a fall risk assessment was completed, interventions were implemented (such as bed alarms or side rails), and the patient was educated about calling for assistance, this can provide evidence that you met the standard of care.

Charting Practices That Can Protect You in Court

Proper documentation is your best defense in legal proceedings. Here are the essential charting practices that can protect you if your documentation is scrutinized in a lawsuit.

1. Document Every Patient Interaction

Every patient interaction—whether it involves assessments, interventions, or education—should be documented thoroughly. Even seemingly minor actions, such as assisting a patient with ambulation or educating them about medication side effects, should be recorded. These small details can become critical pieces of evidence in a lawsuit.

Example: If a patient claims they were not adequately educated about the risks of a procedure, your documentation of the education you provided, including specific details about what was discussed, can serve as proof that you met your obligations.

2. Be Objective, Not Subjective

Avoid using subjective or emotional language in your documentation. Instead, focus on objective, factual descriptions of what you observed, what actions you took, and how the patient responded. Subjective language, such as "patient was difficult" or "patient seemed upset," is open to interpretation and can be misused in legal proceedings.

Example: Instead of writing, "The patient was upset," document the specific behaviors: "Patient raised their voice and refused to take prescribed medication after explanation of potential side effects."

3. Document Changes in the Patient's Condition

One of the most common reasons for litigation is failure to monitor or respond to changes in a patient's condition. It's critical to document any changes, no matter how minor, and your subsequent actions, such as notifying the physician or initiating new interventions.

Example: If a patient develops shortness of breath, document the onset of symptoms, your assessment (e.g., vital signs, lung sounds), communication with the physician, and any treatments administered (e.g., oxygen therapy).

4. Use Proper Abbreviations and Terminology

Only use facility-approved abbreviations and terminology. Ambiguous abbreviations can lead to misunderstandings in court. For example, "QD" (once daily) can be misread as "QID" (four times daily), leading to potential confusion about medication administration. When in doubt, spell out terms fully.

5. Document Communication with the Healthcare Team

Communication with physicians, specialists, and other healthcare team members is crucial in providing comprehensive care. It's equally important to document these communications, especially when they involve changes to the treatment plan or reporting significant changes in the patient's condition.

Example: If you report a patient's abnormal vital signs to a physician and receive new orders, document the time of the communication, what was discussed, and the orders received. This ensures that there is a clear record of the care plan and the collaboration between team members.

6. Avoid Altering or Backdating Documentation

Altering or backdating entries is not only unethical but also illegal. If an error is discovered in your documentation, follow your facility's policy for making corrections, which typically involves adding an addendum with the current date and explaining why the correction is needed. Never attempt to conceal mistakes by altering the original record.

Example: If you realize you forgot to document a medication administration, make a late entry that clearly states, "Late entry: Administered 5 mg morphine IV at 2:00 PM for pain rated at 7/10."

Responding When Your Documentation is Called into Question

Despite your best efforts, there may be times when your documentation is called into question during an investigation or lawsuit. Here's what to do if that happens:

1. Remain Calm and Professional

It's natural to feel anxious if your documentation is being scrutinized in a legal setting, but it's important to remain calm and professional. Stick to the facts and avoid becoming defensive. If you are asked to testify or provide a statement about your documentation, be honest and straightforward.

2. Review Your Documentation Carefully

Before responding to questions about your documentation, take the time to review your notes carefully. This will help you refresh your memory about the care you provided and ensure that you're fully prepared to answer questions accurately.

3. Be Honest About Mistakes

If mistakes or omissions are identified in your documentation, be transparent about them. Explain any relevant circumstances that may have contributed to the error (e.g., a particularly busy shift or an emergency situation), but never attempt to cover up or minimize the mistake.

4. Seek Legal Counsel

If your documentation is part of a lawsuit or investigation, seek legal counsel. An attorney who specializes in healthcare law can guide you through the process and help you navigate any questions about your charting. They can also advise you on how to protect your professional reputation and license.

Defensive documentation is more than just a strategy for providing high-quality patient care—it is a critical safeguard for your professional practice. By maintaining thorough, accurate, and objective records, you can protect yourself in the event of litigation and demonstrate that you provided care in accordance with the standards of nursing practice. In the next chapter, we'll explore the importance of maintaining patient confidentiality in documentation, including how to comply with HIPAA regulations and protect sensitive information from unauthorized access.

Chapter 10

Continuous Improvement: Ongoing Education and Best Practices in Documentation

In today's fast-paced and technology-driven healthcare environment, nurses must continuously evolve their skills, particularly in documentation, to ensure that they meet changing regulatory requirements, legal standards, and technological advancements. Proper documentation serves as the backbone of nursing practice, ensuring patient safety, legal protection, and quality care. However, keeping documentation practices current and compliant requires ongoing learning, self-assessment, and adaptation to new systems. In this chapter, we will dive deeply into the importance of staying updated with regulations, how to incorporate chart audits and self-reviews into daily practice, and provide a wealth of resources for continuous learning and professional development.

Keeping Up-to-Date with Changing Regulations and Technology

1. Evolving Regulatory Requirements

Healthcare regulations are not static—they evolve in response to technological advancements, emerging healthcare challenges, and shifts in patient care protocols. For nurses, this means continuously adapting to updated guidelines issued by regulatory bodies such as the Centers for Medicare & Medicaid Services (CMS), the Joint Commission, and state Boards of Nursing. Adherence to these regulations is crucial not only for patient safety but also for protecting a nurse's license and ensuring compliance with audits and investigations.

Example: Updates to HIPAA (Health Insurance Portability and Accountability Act) over the years have included stricter guidelines on how patient information should be shared and documented electronically. A nurse who is unaware of these updates may inadvertently violate patient privacy, leading to penalties or even license suspension.

How to Stay Informed:

Follow Key Regulatory Agencies: Regularly visit the websites of CMS, state nursing boards, and the Joint Commission. These agencies frequently publish updates, guidelines, and clarifications about documentation standards.

Subscribe to Newsletters: Many professional organizations, such as the American Nurses Association (ANA) and the National Council of State Boards of Nursing (NCSBN), offer free newsletters and webinars that keep members updated on legal changes affecting documentation.

Employer-Sponsored Education: Healthcare organizations often hold seminars or in-service training sessions on regulatory changes and compliance. Participating in these sessions is an efficient way to stay current without having to seek out external resources.

2. Advancements in Documentation Technology

The rapid adoption of Electronic Health Records (EHRs) has transformed how nurses document patient care. While EHRs offer numerous benefits, including improved accessibility, reduced errors, and better data integration, they also present challenges. Nurses must continuously develop their skills to use EHRs effectively while avoiding common pitfalls such as over-reliance on templates or overlooking critical patient details due to automation.

EHRs and Technology Trends:

Cloud-Based and Mobile EHR Systems: Many healthcare facilities are transitioning to cloud-based EHR systems that allow secure access from multiple devices, including mobile phones and tablets. Nurses who are adept at navigating these platforms can document in real-time, improving the accuracy and timeliness of their entries.

Interoperability: Healthcare providers are increasingly focusing on interoperability, where different systems across various departments and institutions can communicate seamlessly. Nurses must ensure that documentation aligns across platforms, especially in multi-disciplinary teams or when patients are transferred between facilities.

How to Stay Updated with EHR Advancements:

Ongoing Training: EHR systems frequently update their interfaces and features. Regular training sessions, provided by the healthcare facility or EHR vendors, help nurses learn new functionalities and best practices. Many EHR providers offer online tutorials and certification courses to enhance proficiency.

Leverage Peer Learning: Peer mentorship is invaluable in mastering EHR systems. Nurses who are comfortable with technology can share tips and strategies for streamlining documentation tasks, minimizing errors, and enhancing workflow efficiency.

Incorporating Chart Audits and Self-Reviews into Daily Practice

The key to maintaining compliant documentation isn't waiting for an external audit—it's embedding a culture of self-audit and continuous improvement in your daily practice. Chart audits and self-reviews offer opportunities to assess and improve documentation before it comes under scrutiny by external auditors or during an investigation.

1. Understanding Chart Audits

Chart audits are formal reviews of patient records, typically performed to ensure that documentation adheres to established standards and regulatory requirements. These audits may be internal (conducted by the facility's compliance team) or external (carried out by regulators like CMS or state nursing boards). Regular audits help identify gaps in documentation, areas of non-compliance, and potential risks.

Benefits of Chart Audits:

Improved Quality of Care: Audits help highlight areas where documentation can be improved, ensuring that future patient care plans are clear, concise, and effective.

Legal Protection: Regularly auditing charts allows nurses and institutions to identify and correct documentation errors before they become the subject of legal disputes or regulatory scrutiny.

Early Detection of Systemic Issues: If audit results reveal consistent documentation errors across departments or units, the facility can implement systemic changes to improve compliance and prevent widespread issues.

How to Participate in Chart Audits:

Volunteer for Peer Reviews: Participating in peer-to-peer chart reviews allows nurses to review each other's documentation practices, offering feedback while learning from the practices of others.

Use Automated Audit Tools: Many EHR systems have built-in tools that can automatically flag incomplete or inconsistent documentation. Nurses can use these tools to self-audit their records in real-time and address any issues immediately.

2. Self-Reviews and Best Practices

A culture of self-review helps ensure that nursing documentation is complete, accurate, and timely. Conducting routine self-reviews—either daily or weekly—can prevent errors from accumulating over time and reduce the need for time-consuming corrections later.

Steps for Effective Self-Review:

Use Checklists: Create a checklist that mirrors regulatory requirements and best practices for your specific unit or specialty. For instance, a checklist for post-operative care might include items like pain management assessments, wound care documentation, and patient education.

Assess for Completeness: Verify that each entry in the patient's chart is complete. For instance, if documenting a medication administration, ensure that it includes the dosage, time of administration, patient's reaction, and any follow-up.

Check for Timeliness: Review timestamps and ensure that documentation is entered as close to the time of the intervention as possible. Late entries should be properly labeled and explained according to your facility's guidelines.

Seek Peer Feedback: Engaging in informal peer reviews allows nurses to receive constructive criticism from colleagues, offering fresh perspectives on areas that need improvement.

Resources for Further Learning and Professional Development in Charting

Nurses committed to improving their documentation skills must embrace lifelong learning. There is an abundance of resources available to help nurses refine their charting practices, stay up-to-date with evolving standards, and enhance their professional development.

1. Professional Organizations and Certifications

Joining a professional nursing organization provides access to numerous resources, including publications, continuing education opportunities, and networking with peers who share similar professional interests.

American Nurses Association (ANA): ANA offers comprehensive resources on legal issues, documentation best practices, and continuing education courses designed to keep nurses up-to-date with changes in healthcare regulations.

National Association of Healthcare Quality (NAHQ): NAHQ provides resources for quality improvement in healthcare, including best practices for documentation that aligns with quality standards and compliance regulations.

Specialized Certifications: Certifications such as the Certified Professional in Healthcare Quality (CPHQ) or Certified Documentation Improvement Practitioner (CDIP) provide in-depth training on documentation standards, quality improvement, and legal protection.

2. Online Learning Platforms and Continuing Education

Online platforms make it easy for nurses to access continuing education courses on documentation from the comfort of their homes or during their work breaks. Many courses are self-paced and can be completed as time allows.

Medscape: Medscape offers free CEUs on a wide variety of topics, including nursing documentation, compliance, and legal issues.

Nurse.com: Nurse.com provides affordable online courses that focus on improving nursing documentation, addressing both clinical and legal aspects.

State Nursing Boards: Many state nursing boards provide lists of approved continuing education courses specifically designed to meet state requirements for license renewal, often including documentation best practices.

3. Mentorship and Peer Learning

Experienced nurses can offer valuable insights into documentation practices. A strong mentorship relationship allows less experienced nurses to learn from seasoned professionals who understand both the clinical and legal implications of documentation.

Mentorship Programs: Many hospitals and healthcare institutions offer formal mentorship programs where new nurses are paired with veteran nurses. These programs are great opportunities to discuss documentation challenges, ask questions, and get real-time feedback.

Peer Support Groups: Establishing a peer support group within your unit can foster open discussions about documentation issues, provide solutions to common challenges, and build a culture of continuous improvement.

Incorporating continuous improvement into your documentation practice is not just a legal and ethical obligation; it is a crucial part of delivering high-quality patient care. By staying current with regulatory changes, actively participating in chart audits and self-reviews, and taking advantage of the vast resources available for professional development, you ensure that your documentation reflects the best possible standard of nursing practice.

Moving forward, embracing lifelong learning and seeking out opportunities to refine your skills will keep your documentation compliant, comprehensive, and ready to withstand the scrutiny of audits, investigations, or legal challenges. As healthcare regulations and technologies evolve, so too must your approach to documentation.

CONCLUSION

As a registered nurse, charting is not just a daily task—it's a critical aspect of your practice that safeguards your career and ensures patient safety. Accurate, timely, and thorough documentation is the backbone of your professional integrity. It protects you from legal and regulatory scrutiny and demonstrates your commitment to providing quality care.

Nurses are increasingly facing scrutiny from regulatory boards, legal teams, and healthcare administrators. Inadequate or incomplete charting can result in disciplinary actions, legal battles, and even the suspension or loss of your nursing license. However, by mastering the art of comprehensive documentation, you not only shield yourself from such risks but also enhance your value as a healthcare professional. Clear, concise, and complete charting allows for seamless communication among the healthcare team, ensuring that patient care is delivered efficiently and without error.

In addition to protecting your license, accurate documentation serves as a valuable record for patient care continuity. It enables other healthcare providers to pick up where you left off, ensuring that the patient's history, medications, interventions, and outcomes are well-documented.

Bonus Tips for Charting on a Typical Shift

Chart in Real-Time: Whenever possible, chart immediately after a patient interaction. Delaying documentation can lead to forgotten details and potential errors.

Be Objective and Specific: Avoid subjective language. Instead of writing "patient seems better," document concrete observations, such as "patient reports a pain level of 4/10, down from 8/10, after administration of morphine."

Follow Facility Protocols: Every healthcare facility has specific guidelines for documentation. Make sure you're familiar with these policies and adhere to them.

Use Approved Abbreviations Only: Avoid using personal shorthand that could be misinterpreted. Stick to your facility's approved abbreviations and terminology.

Document All Communications: If you report a change in a patient's condition to a physician or another healthcare professional, document the communication and any instructions or orders received.

Cover All Bases with Incident Reporting: In the event of an incident (e.g., a fall, medication error), ensure that your charting is accurate, factual, and devoid of personal opinions. Use the incident reporting system according to your facility's protocols.

Time Your Entries: Every note should include the time of the action or observation, not just when you happen to chart it. This provides an accurate timeline for patient care.

End Your Shift with a Review: Before handing off to the next nurse or ending your shift, review your notes to ensure nothing was missed.

Consistency in end-of-shift charting improves care continuity and reduces errors.

By integrating these strategies into your daily routine, you enhance the quality of your patient care while also protecting your most valuable asset—your nursing license. Accurate and timely charting is the hallmark of a responsible, professional nurse and is critical to both patient outcomes and career longevity.

www.ingramcontent.com/pod-product-compliance
Lightning Source LLC
Chambersburg PA
CBHW070126230526
45472CB00004B/1437